Psychedelic Experience For Personal Benefit

Psychedelic Experience For Personal Benefit

Robert E. Leihy

To order additional copies of this book, contact:
Xlibris Corporation
1-888-795-4274
www.Xlibris.com
Orders@Xlibris.com
130181

Contents

This book is dedicated to my mentor,
Dr. Stanislav Grof

Author's Note

This essay is careful not to advocate the use of psychedelic drugs but to describe their effects, their possible uses, their safety, and cautions to be taken in their use.

The general thrust of the essay is to show how psychedelics, including mild marijuana, can be used as occasional low-dose "training aids" to guide oneself in the practice of deeper tranquility, physical well-being, cool rationality, and creativity. Since marijuana is becoming more legal, it is no longer necessary to be a subject in a research program to take advantage of the psychedelic experience for personal exploration. The essay also describes some aspects of the high-dose cosmic and religious experiences and how to resolve conflicts that are sometimes found on that level of abstraction.

Psychedelic drugs, as a class, have been found to have significant beneficial uses. For instance, MDMA has been found to help treat posttraumatic stress disorder and marijuana has been found to reduce the symptoms of chemotherapy. Being the largest cash crop in the United States ($35 billion), marijuana is clearly useful in safely satisfying the high demand for diversion and "self transcendence" that exists in all cultures. For some, psychedelic drugs can also be a stimulation of religious concepts and points of view and in this sense they could be considered as sacramental.

After over 50 years of exposure to the area, I personally have not heard of a single case of violence, inappropriate sexual behavior, or even a car accident attributable specifically to the psychedelic experience itself. The major effects of psychedelics are relaxation, meditation, and creativity. The various synthetic and naturally occuring psychedelic drugs are absolutely non-toxic and non-addicting. Beside their usefulness, they appear to be statistically extremely safe.

The high demand for drug-induced diversion and self transcendence is world-wide and has existed throughout history. Overuse of these drugs, including alcohol, has led to much tragedy as exemplified by the myth of the mermaids who lured sailors to crash their ships onto the rocky shores. To the extent that safe psychedelics can satisfy this demand, they will be a blessing. A few preliminary findings already indicate that alcohol abuse and crime in general are reduced in neighborhoods that have medical marijuana distribution points.

Satisfactory levels of deep tranquility can be cultivated with or without any drugs at all, and practicing to achieve them is a meaningful challenge and satisfying lifestyle. Many have done so and are doing so. These states can be used as natural escapes from the turbulence, stress, and tedium of daily life and at the same time can provide the pleasure and satisfactions associated with them. Psychedelic drugs can safely and easily reveal some of the deeper levels of positive experience that are possible and thereby facilitate the practice. They can also be used to stimulate penetrating meditation on ways to resolve tension issues that block the path to tranquility.

In the past, psychedelic drug research has usually involved a low number of high-dose sessions. These have been found to be of value and they are very interesting, but when they are over they are over. In addition, they are very abstract in nature and not easy to remember or to put into practice in daily life. The insights gained in lower and moderate doses are much easier to remember and to practice, cultivate, and customize in daily life. In addition, the lower dose sessions can more easily be guided into chosen topics.

For instance, a person might discover a deeper physical relaxation and a deeper peace of mind during a psychedelic session. If he were to practice that state of being during daily life and perhaps during future psychedelic sessions, it could become more and more of a part of his personality. He would know that such experiences exists within himself and that they can be a targets to aim for and to cultivate. A known target can help to organize mental forces that otherwise might remain dispersed. As will be shown, there are many other states of being, useful personal insights, and productive attitudes that are often revealed by expanded consciousness that can become cultivated and customized as parts of daily life.

The "training aid" approach to the use of psychedelic drugs could be used, within reason, by people at all levels of mental maturity. Even well-adjusted fully-functioning people have plenty of room to explore in such areas as the philosophical and the religious. People who already use a psychedelic primarily for diversion and pleasure could continue to do so but to add a dimension of personal benefit to their experiences. This technique could also be combined with conventional psychotherapy if so desired. There would more material to work with, it would emerge by itself, and both goals and blocks to progress would become more vivid. Because psychedelics can be used very effectively to help train the body in deep relaxation, I am guessing that psychotherapeutic techniques similar to systematic desensitization would be effective in the treatment of phobias and similar tension issues. Since the psychedelic experience tends to be somewhat euphoric on the average, formal psychotherapy as well as personal growth can become both pleasant as well as useful and interesting.

I have been involved in the relatively new field of psychedelic drug research for much of my adult life, both professionally as a psychotherapist and also casually as an interested explorer. I have had the privilege of acting as "ground control" for well over two hundred people experiencing high dose LSD sessions: normal volunteers, mental patients, and alcoholics. Over time, my colleagues and I have experienced several psychedelic sessions ourselves at low to high dosage levels. I have personally explored these realms of consciousness carefully and thoroughly within myself from both the psychological and the spiritual perspectives with different natural and synthetic psychedelic drugs.

Since psychedelic experience is essentially a stimulation of intuitive thought, low and moderate doses of a psychedelic drug can be used for simple recreation, deep relaxation, deep meditation, self analysis, situational analysis, heightened perception, and expanded consciousness. Higher doses, with a few precautions, can be used to vividly explore cosmic and religious concepts. All of this can be done in the comfort and safety of a recliner without even a hint of a hangover.

Since the statistically safe psychedelic drug marijuana is becoming more accepted and more legal, I think that now would be a good time to describe the structure that I have learned regarding how psychedelics can be harnessed for personal developmenth and benefit in addition to recreation and diversion.

Safety

Perhaps the first and most important point to consider regarding psychedelic drugs, including marijuana, is that in spite of the lingering concern over their safety, the fact remains that the drugs by themselves and the psychedelic experience by itself have proven themselves as being statistically almost perfectly safe. They appear safe mentally, physically, and socially. This is the "elephant in the room" within the controversy. It is an extremely tragic example of a tempest in a teapot considering the violence associated with the production and distribution of marijuana. Between 2006 and 2012, about 60,000 people have died in the Mexican drug wars and many otherwise innocent people have been jailed and their lives ruined. This scenario may one day be considered as one of the most cruel and deadly fiascos in history.

These drugs by themselves are not addicting or toxic and they lead only to calm stimulated meditation or the enjoyment of low key but vivid artistic or creative activities.

After fifty years of experience I have yet to hear or read about a single case of violence or sexual misconduct attributable exclusively to marijuana or any other psychedelic drug by itself. This is certainly not the case with alcohol or meth.

There are plenty of problems involving corruption and violence in the production and the distribution of marijuana because it is classified as illegal by the federal government. One reason that the demand for marijuana is high is because people recognize that it is the one safe drug that can be used for "self transcendence" as well as for satisfying and useful deep meditation and creative activities. It can be enjoyed by the same people who put high premiums on personal health and social standing because these attributes are not affected negatively as is the case with too much alcohol or meth. Marijuana is in reality a safe, useful, and valuable commodity in high demand, and different people and different factions of people would very much like to control it and make money on it. I expect that eventually enough people will become convinced of its safety and that it will be legalized and bought and sold like any other commodity with only minor restrictions associated with it. It offers pleasure, education, better functioning, better health, and safety all at the same time so I doubt that it will be needlessly suppressed forever.

In his book *Marijuana Is Safer So Why Are We Driving People To Drink?* Steve Fox describes in detail and with many references the social and legal forces that encourage the overuse of dangerous and deadly alcohol and the suppression of the much safer marijuana.

The "reefer madness" myth was a complete hoax, but its name suggests a possibility that might give pause under certain circumstances. An occasional insight, inspiration, emotion, intuition, or fantasy springing to mind might not be the least bit threatening to a person, but a constant upwelling flow of such material could possibly be interpreted as something invading and overwhelming consciousness. If a totally inexperienced person should accidentally take a high dose of a psychedelic drug without knowing what to expect, this could be so threatening that it could be interpreted as madness. None of my totally inexperienced high dose clients felt the least bit threatened as their psychedelic experience took effect, but they were well prepared verbally and knew exactly what to expect. Once a person realizes that the rational mind can stay intact right along with the upwelling intuitive material during a psychedelic experience, it seems interesting rather than threatening. In fact, when dosage is such that the rational and the intuitive sides of the mind can work in conjunction with each other, deep penetration into chosen topics is possible. The rational mind can think clearly while the intuitive mind can occasionally and unexpectedly float useful insights up to consciousness along with the other psychedelic material.

The fact that psychedelic drugs are also classified as "hallucinogenic" could also give pause. The fact is that the hallucinations can more accurately be described as amplifications of the process where faces and animals are seen in clouds and in the embers of a fire. It is interesting to watch them change and they can be blinked away. There is never anything as vivid as a solid object, but an oriental carpet can become a beautiful kaleidoscope of changing colors and patterns. The faces in photographs can change identity and mood. I consider these visual amplifications as representations of the fact that the intuitive mind is very good at clustering data and presenting it in symbolic form to consciousness. This capability of the intuitive mind is very useful during meditation and self-analysis and is discussed later. Inner visual imagery is often quite vivid, but it goes away when the eyes are opened.

Overdoses of psychedelics are extremely rare and probably accidental. They lead to nothing but deeper meditation for longer periods of time. There will never be rehabilitation clinics for overdoses or addictions to psychedelics. Assuming that a person can accurately choose his own dosage, different comfort levels can be selected for the purposes of recreation, meditation, or the exploration of the cosmic and religious abstractions.

After not having any psychedelic experiences at all for a period of about thirty years, I initially got an accidental huge overdose of a marijuana pastry. The young saleslady at the medical marijuana distribution center told me that one brownie was equal to one dose. Later I found out that it was equal to four doses. The brownie caused complete couchlock for about four hours, but I had no trouble whatsoever with the experience itself because I was already familiar with how to handle high doses. The overdose experience did not seem much different from a regular high dose experience. I just let it flow by. My rational mind was still always present when so desired. At the end of the experience there was not even a hint of a hangover and I felt better than ever. This indicates that overdoses of psychedelics are not necessarily bad trips, that they won't kill you, and that they won't drive you crazy. I am quite sure that there will never be rehabilitation clinics for addictions to psychedelics or hospitalizations for overdoses.

Without going into details, I am guessing that experiences of this nature with the proper dosage of a psychedelic drug might very well substitute for the binge drinking of alcohol. The extreme self-transcendence and the escape from the world would certainly be there, but instead of damage to health and social standing and a long and unpleasant sick guilty hangover, there would be something pleasant, interesting, spiritually gratifying,and actually psychotherapeutic. Hopefully such a substitution will be found to be possible in the future.

On the basis of my own experience and that of people who I have known, frequency of use of psychedelics tends to diminish over time. The relaxation, introspection, abstract levels of thought, and creativity that they offer come more naturally. Eventually, occasional low-dose sessions tend to become "short vacations" as well as reinforcement of what has already been learned.

Cautions

One caution to be considered is that short term memory is affected because new mental material is continually flowing to consciousness. It is easy to leave something cooking on the stove or to be distracted while driving. Any kind of risky activity should be avoided, as is true with any mind-altering drug including alcohol.

There are two significant cautions to be observed with high dose experiences. One is that it can become possible to mix up the contents of the mental inner world with the real outer world. The reason that this can take place is because the mind is a single virtual image filling a single awareness. It contains what appears to be a representation of an external reality as well as an internal mental world. The main difference between the two is the complete flexibility of the inner world. If something in the inner world becomes vivid enough, it can appear as being part of the external world and the two can become mixed together. It is for this reason that it is probably safest to experience a high dose in a recliner or on a couch rather than being involved in complexities relating to the outer world. An extreme example would be where in the inner world a person dreams that he can soar freely through space while in the real world he is near an open window. For this reason, it is very highly recommended that a person choosing a high dose experience should have an experienced companion nearby to provide a solid rational platform in the real outside world. Knowing that "ground control" is present to take care of any real-world problems that might arise also allows a person to let go and become completely involved with the inner world.

While considering this point of view, one might devote some energy into meditating on how to improve the nature of the part of his mind that represents his body and the outside world. In figuring out how to make improvements and then putting them into practice, within the constraints of natural law, of course, he is not only improving the quality of his inner mental existence but also that of the apparent outside material world.

There are many interesting ramifications to the point of view that we live entirely in our minds.

The other significant caution is the possibility of a "bad trip". I am quite sure that this is most likely to happen when an inexperienced person takes a high dose under bad conditions or without verbal preparation. No doubt it is even more likely if that person has had a hard life. None of my high-dose clients had bad trips but they were well prepared verbally beforehand. Since the high dose experience evokes cosmic concepts, I discuss some ways to handle high-dose bad trips in the later chapter called "Managing Bad Trips". Some of the cosmic concepts naturally have grim components, such as the fact of suffering in the human condition, the paranoid point of view, and various definitions of the afterlife, but they can all be explored from the standpoint of a calm rational student-scientist without being overwhelmed by them. An experienced "ground control" can hold a rational conversation with the student-scientist at these times and the two can verbally examine and possibly interpret parts of the experience as it flows by.

The Nature Of
The Psychedelic Experience

The Stimulated Intuitive Mind

The physical nature of the psychedelic experience is generally one of relaxation and blissful feelings. The mental side can generally be conceptualized as the stimulation of the intuitive side of the mind. In the model that I like to use, the intuitive side clusters new insights while what I call the "spontaneous thought generator" converts them to rational forms that can be remembered or communicated. We have all had insights that take a little time to put into words. In normal daily consciousness these insights are what are often called the "aha" insights that pop to mind when completely unexpected as does other creative material. During psychedelic experience, the output of the intuitive mind flows to consciousness on a continuous basis and takes various forms such as words, visual symbols, music, feelings, and what I like to call "appreciations".

The intuitive part of the mind that puts together spontaneous insights works outside of awareness and it obviously processes real-world data. Since it produces something new that we have never even thought of, it is smarter in some ways than we are up here in our normal rational minds. These insights are almost always useful and to our benefit, suggesting that the intuitive mind is a silent inner ally who is on our side and who is just as interested in our survival and well-being as we are. Sometimes these insights are minor, sometimes they are more general, and sometimes they are more like sweeping revelations. Sometimes the broader concepts that come to mind take quite a bit of time to "clothe" adequately in words or other symbols. No doubt many people will be happy to find out that their inner self is not necessarily filled with repressed antisocial impulses, as has been suggested in the past.

The rational mind can watch the intuitive material emerge, get as deeply involved with it as desired, and then come back out again. With higher doses it becomes possible to become almost totally involved with the various aspects of the experience. Relating to everyday levels of abstraction takes place with low dosages, more sweeping mythical and archetypal abstractions at moderate levels, and cosmic and religious abstractions with high dosages. There is plenty of territory in between, one interesting area being that of self-reflection, situational analysis, and personal growth.

Sometimes when reviewing a new insight, it is clear that the intuitive side of the mind can process strictly intuitive information such as subtle impressions, connections between multiple events, and underlying influences in addition to individual events at the more concrete level. It also has an excellent memory. It can remember the expressions on people's faces, nuances of gestures, and background influences as it clusters information for new insights to be formulated and presented to consciousness. Dr. Stanislav Grof (stanislavgrof.com), my mentor, refers to these clusters as COEX (condensed experience) systems.

During moderate and higher doses, the intuitive material of psychedelic experience tends to flow to mind constantly with each new insight or impression quickly replacing the previous one. Some people interpret this as a loss of short term memory, which in a way it is, but I think it is more like water flowing under a bridge. These are good times to have a handheld voice recorder handy. But even if an insight might be lost downstream, it will be found to still be intact if it is revisited later because the work of clustering it together has already been done. It is difficult to backtrack a psychedelic experience, but sometimes it is possible to remember something farther back and then to work forward.

This flow of mental experience, however it is conceptualized or whatever its source is conceptualized to be, is a clear reality during psychedelic experience. The higher the dosage, the more vivid and abstract it becomes. A peaceful mind in a relaxed body can watch and listen as this mental material spontaneously flows up to consciousness.

The intuitive mind can be legitimately conceptualized as a source of pre-existing information and also a plastic mental domain where new ideas, concepts, and attitudes can be planted and cultivated. This cultivation can take place with or without psychedelic stimulation, but the psychedelic stimulation makes the process more vivid and I am assuming faster.

The intuitive mind is obviously aware of the outside world because it spontaneously produces insights with reference to it. So it is always back there silently learning new things from it just as is the rational mind.

Expanded Consciousness

A stimulated intuitive mind works in terms of broader and more global levels of abstraction. Doing so has the advantage of including more factors and data into each concept. It is a less limited way of looking at things. Better decisions scan be made at the broader levels of abstraction because bigger pictures are dealt with. The higher the dosage of the psychedelic drug, the more data is included in each thought and concept that comes to mind. At lower dosages, real-world events are clustered into wholenesses. Instead of considering how one person might have been influential in the rush to war with Iraq, a broader "hysterical epidemic" might be contemplated as being behind it. At moderate dosages, more sweeping concepts such as trends, influences, personalities, archetypes, and myths come to mind. One might consider the concept of charity itself rather than a single charitable act by itself. At high dosages cosmic and religious concepts are considered. One might consider the concept of infinite eternal all-pervading space or of all-pervading spirit, or of stationary eternal time as well as time defined by objects moving in space.

Enhanced Perception

Aldous Huxley (en.wikipedia.org/wiki/The_Doors_of_Perception) describes enhanced perception in his book "Doors of Perception". Authors and gurus who describe this experience, such as Osho at osho.com often state that it is necessary to quiet the rational mind so completely that full attention can be placed onto perception itself. All preconceptions, interpretations, classifications,and judgments need to be temporarily suspended. During psychedelic experience, however, it seems that the beauty and the purity of enhanced perception is strong enough that it can coexist comfortably with the rational mind. It is another example of the intuitive and the rational minds working together. An example would be the poet who converts impressions into words. It is like being totally involved in the perceptual experience while at the same time the rational mind can "skitter" over the surface. The world is perceived as being more vivid and awesome and as such it elicits stronger feeling-impression sensitivities. Every nerve can seem to reverberate with the vibrations of music. The beauty of nature can become breathtaking. Food can become ambrosia. The most absurd and trivial can become miraculous. A blade of grass can be seen to share the same miracle of existence as the entire universe. Works of fine art can literally blaze with the skill and sensitivity of extremely talented people. A person feels that he is seeing "the which of which there is no whicher" or "where it is really at". Some call it "direct perception" while others refer to it as getting "hung up" on something. In our scientific industrialized intellectual culture it is probably the children, the artists, and the musicians who perceive the world from this perspective the best. Being deeply relaxed while enjoying direct perception in the here-and-now moment can be extremely refreshing.

Words and other symbols can be conceptualized as a net that is cast over reality to describe it. These symbols are extremely useful. It is easier to move a mountain or fly to the moon with words rather in the physical world. However, they can also act as a mask for outside reality. The only time that outside reality can shine through the symbolic overlay is when something cannot be described in words. Overlooks to Yosemite Valley in California would be an example. With psychedelics, the awesome quality of the rest of existence can also become more apparent because the miracle and the mystery of how it emerged or is emerging from nothingness can become more vivid.

Self Analysis

At the right moderate dosage level, a person can harness the rational and the intuitive sides of his mind together to meditate deeply and to analyze chosen topics. With each broader level of abstraction, there can be many new insights because of the different points of view. For instance, instead of considering a single event in a person's life, a larger picture might be formed including the setting, previous influences, motivations, purposes, personalities, sensitivities, and the resulting outcomes. A fuller and more vivid picture can emerge. It becomes possible to sense and recognize where any tension issues, disconnects, and misunderstandings might have taken place and how they could be avoided or blocked in future similar situations. Productive actions can be noted more vividly. It is also possible to take advantage of this feature of psychedelic drugs to do a more in-depth analysis of current situations.

Such insights are almost always completely authentic since the intuitive mind works with real-world data, and they provide valuable information on how to help relate more smoothly to the outside world. Volumes could be written on psychotherapy, self-analysis, and situational analysis involving the rational and the intuitive sides of the mind working together. With practice, this process can become something like a team effort with two heads working on the same problem.

An analogy to this process would be sitting in a room facing two radios. THe one on the right could represent the rational mind and the one on the left the intuitive mind. They can take turns producing information. Sometimes they are in sync and producing exactly the same information. This is when they are working together as a third mental entity.

Discovering the mental tension issues that block the path to tranquility is quite easy. All that is necessary is to practice relaxation and see what gets in the way. With a psychedelic, it is usually quite clear what the block is composed of since the intuitive mind tends to cluster topics into meaningful wholenesses. The task becomes to work on the block while it is present in consciousness. Resolutions are sometimes very satisfying "aha" insights. Sometimes they are more vague or general in nature and may require further work. Resolutions to complex problems can be meditated upon with the rational mind while at the same time answers and partial answers can sometimes be provided by the intuitive mind. Some resolutions might be new attitudes or ways of looking at things while others might be physical solutions to real-world problems. Just as it is possible to learn and practice this type of meditation, it is possible to learn and practice deep tranquility and to move back and forth between the two at will.

Neuroplastic Space

MRI research has shown that religious monks who meditate for long periods of time on compassion for the human condition stimulate activity in specific areas of their brains. I believe that with psychedelic stimulation a person can relatively quickly do something similar. It is possible to conceptualize, cultivate, and meditate upon chosen ideal concept-images in "neuroplastic space" that in turn can become pervasive central influences on one's entire personality. I have no idea how these images work on the neural level; they may simply be newly activated memory networks, but they do in fact work and they can influence daily life in positive directions. For instance, during psychedelic experience a person might meditate on periods of deep serenity, patience, and acceptance and willfully associate them with mental images of something such as Buddha images. The influences of these images will automatically pop to mind and to help him to keep calm when stressful situations arise in daily life. These images can be remembered and cultivated even in normal daily consciousness and can act as self-constructed guiding lights through the maze of life. I am quite sure that the cultivation of these images could replace unwanted habits. The surprisingly extreme influence these images can have is described in my later section called "Neuroplastic Influence". These images can become very vivid during psychedelic experience, and since they are self-chosen and good it is a pleasure to work with them and to develop them.

A study of women becoming nuns, another of people who had won the lottery, and perhaps others have indicated that changes in circumstances often have little long-lasting effects on baseline mood and approaches to life. To the extent to which this is true, such changes might better be made on the inside. I believe that this is possible through the discovery and cultivation of neuroplastic images and that occasional low-dose psychedelic experiences can facilitate the process.

Rational Imagery

In the model that I like to use, the intuitive mind works outside of awareness and in this sense it is invisible and silent. When it has clustered an insight, it sends it to the spontaneous thought generator where it is converted into some kind of rational form that can be remembered or communicated to the outside world. The conversion process could be interpreted as the psychedelic experience itself. It can include words, images, insights, general understandings, emotional feelings and what I like to call "appreciations". The flow of this material can be fascinating to say the least. With moderate and high doses it usually flows by rather steadily and constantly, so it is not always easy to present it to the outside world as it happens. Authors, poets, and people interested in personal growth would no doubt benefit from handheld voice recorders at these times. Musicians would have their instruments and recorders handy. There is a story about an artist who vowed to paint his visual imagery during his psychedelic experience but who got caught up in a single dot and had to paint later from memory.

It is not a mystery why creative people often state that they are merely the messengers of what they produce because so much of it emerges spontaneously. To be noted is that a certain percentage of the psychedelic experience is pretty much strictly on the "feeling" or "appreciation" level and that realistic, geometric, or organic visual imagery is the only medium that can interpret it. Sometimes there is no rational interpretation at all, and just the feelings and the impressions flow by.

The Inner Voice

Since we normally think in words, we actually hear an inner voice much of the time. Even in normal daily consciousness, however, we can imagine that we are talking to someone else. With psychedelic stimulation, this "someone else" can become quite vivid and independent. Carl Jung refers to "autonomous complexes" where the mind can temporarily construct entire second mental personalities that can be related to in the inner world. Although common in dreams, this process can come as quite a surprise the first time it is experienced in a psychedelic session. For psychedelic experience, I like the concept of a single spontaneous thought generator that can shape-change as appropriate for what is being communicated and experienced at the moment.

As the level of abstraction increases with dosage, there can be a flow of new insights on those levels because of the new points of view. Often these insights pop to mind in verbal form. When this is done, there can be the impression that an "inner teacher" is communicating with the rational mind. In this way the spontaneous thought generator can become personified. It can take on the role associated with the information being communicated. On the low level of abstraction, it might take on the role of an actual human teacher, on the moderate level it might take on the role of a mythical wizard, and, on the cosmic level, a spirit. Even if a person feels that he is talking with God, he may be "simply" receiving insights regarding cosmic and religious concepts as the intuitive mind clusters extremely general abstractions and presents them to consciousness in a rational form. Of course, it is impossible to prove that it is or is not really really God Himself. In any case, the "teaching" quality of the psychedelic experience has been known for centuries. The spontaneous thought generator can also be conceptualized as a persons' "muse" which can shape-change as the situation calls for. Carlos Castanada's book "The Teachings of Don Juan" deals with this topic. In it, "Mescalito" is considered to be a spiritual teacher that exists within the psychedelic Mescal cactus itself. As will be discussed in a later section on cosmic and religious experience, it is impossible to prove or disprove the existence of spirit or its function. Therefore, no one really knows whether the inner voice is a presentation of spirit or the output of a physical brain, but it can be conceptualized either way with equal ease and as such the question can actually be ignored if so desired.

From the cosmic-materialistic point of view, the galaxies of atoms that make up the drug itself interact with the galaxies of atoms that make up the brain, the combination of the two which in turn miraculously yield something new and meaningful in the immaterial, virtual, three-dimensional image that we call our mind. So even from the materialistic point of view, the new information comes from the drug. From the spiritualistic-materialistic point of view, spirit moves the atoms of the brain in such a way as to create the image. From the strictly spiritual point of view, the entire process is God's dream. While the movement of atoms might be considered as strictly materialistic, awareness and meaning could be considered as being beyond the material and bordering on the spiritual.

Self Transcendence

I like to use the phrase "self-transcendence" to describe the experiences ranging from a pleasant "high" up to the deepest involvement with the broadest of cosmic and spiritual abstractions. They all refer to getting outside of one's everyday self and looking down upon the world from broader mental perspectives while usually feeling expanded, optimistic, and good.

The need for self-transcendence exists in all cultures and varies from person to person. For some people it is so intense that they are willing put their health and their social standing in jeopardy for its sake. Some conceptualize at as a spiritual quest. It can be pursued with a variety of drugs, alcohol probably being the most popular worldwide. Other methods include those suggested by the religions, sensory isolation, holotropic breathwork, fasting, extreme sports and risks, and the identification with crowd mentality at times such as when the home team wins the Super Bowl.

I am guessing that a person who is seeking spiritual transcendence and combining it with the use of alcohol or some other unhealthy stimulant could instead find great gratification with well-aimed high-dose psychedelic sessions instead. He might be able to relate to what he comfortably conceptualized as his own inner concept of God or at the same time as possibly with God Himself. In other words, he would be comfortable with the concept that even though spirit is a mystery he could still enjoy spiritual-psychological benefits such as faith and the identification with the oneness of the universe. All this could be contemplated in a recliner rather than in a gutter. Any other interested person could also explore these same levels of abstraction and no doubt find the same satisfactions. Dr. Walter Pahnke's "Good Friday Experiment" can be researched on the Internet in this regard.

To the best of my knowledge, the safest, easiest, and most satisfying method of self-transcendence in the entire world is with the psychedelic drugs. Not only can they lead to all of the satisfactions mentioned above, but even to the satisfaction of getting "wasted", or temporarily escaping completely from the turmoil, tedium, frustration, uncertainty, and confusion of daily life. As such, I hope and believe that high doses of a safe psychedelic drug can come to replace some of the binge drinking and the extreme overuse of the dangerous and addicting drugs. It would seem that the cosmic revelations associated with the high dose experience could provide some new and positive points of view, as could meditation on current circumstances with lower doses.

I am guessing and hoping that psychedelics could serve the purpose of satisfying the need for self-transcendence in people who would otherwise gravitate toward the more dangerous drugs for the same purpose. In other words, they could act as the opposite of "gateway" drugs. One newspaper article I read said that alcohol use went down in neighborhoods that had a medical marijuana cooperative.

I am sure that psychedelics do not "scratch the same biological itch" that results from the withdrawals from other drugs, but they do at least provide the desired self transcendence. Perhaps for some people that would be enough.

Some of the religious experiences/concepts have already been described, such as melting into a Nirvana of spirit, conceptualizing all-pervading spirit as filling the universe, or seeing the magic of causation unfolding. Experiences of this nature and others like them can be extremely satisfying on a very deep level.

I also believe that the psychedelic drugs can be used by anyone to stimulate levels of focused deep meditation that can reveal better ways of relating to daily life and to lead to more calmness, contentment, peace of mind, and to less of a need to escape from the world at all. The broader concepts at the higher dosages are always there, and they can be explored at leisure if so desired. Knowing that the "spiritual home" concept is within one's being and that it can be experienced again can be very reassuring. Revisiting the broad conceptual levels on occasion would certainly not be a sin, and doing so would be safe. These experiences can help to satisfy the "spiritual quest" in a very positive manner even though it turns out that spirit is a mystery. Finding the path to personal growth can give considerable direction and satisfaction in life.

Practicing contentment leads to more contentment while escaping from discontent, especially with dangerous drugs, results in returns to the same level of discontent and possibly to circumstances that are even worse. It is far more productive to mentally water the flowers and to let the weeds dry up rather than to hide from the weeds and return to them repeatedly. A positive and constructive outlook on the world is certainly the desirable way to see things and it is worth working toward.

I am quite sure that the story about sailors being seduced by the songs of mermaids to crash on the rocks is meant to be an analogy to the desire for self-transcendence by means of alcohol. The story points out that sometimes people risk death for the sake of self transcendence. Perhaps it would make sense to recognize the fact that the need for self-transcendence is an extremely powerful force in society, ranging from a couple of drinks in restaurants to alcohol binges to ravishing one's body with narcotics to hurtling through space on a motorcycle. If this craving for self-transcendence could be satisfied with safe psychedelic drugs in a recliner and if a person could at the same time learn deeper peace of mind and more harmonious relationships with the outside world, it would be a win-win-win situation. All this could take place without even a hint of a hangover or a significant loss of motor control. By analogy, the sailors could find a sandy beach for their longboats and could pursue the exquisite songs of the mermaids without the suffering or the guilt associated with the possible eventual destruction of their lifestyles and their health.

Perhaps one day the pursuit of self-transcendence with a safe psychedelic drug will be regarded as a worthwhile and useful activity rather than just as a degenerative need to get high for the sake of escape and pleasure as it currently is considered with the more dangerous drugs.

The Path To Fulfillment

Fulfillment could be defined as a combination of relating to the world with maximum sensitivity and efficiency while at the same time feeling good. Feeling good is covered in the next section. This is about the best we can do while living in this world of occasional hostility, occasional demands, continuous uncertainty, ultimate incomprehensibility, and an unknown afterlife.

At present most psychedelic research is focused on psychotherapy; in other words, on the resolution of troublesome mental or emotional tensions. But I would like to suggest that psychedelic drugs can also be used to illuminate a path that anyone can take toward greater relaxation and deeper peace of mind.

A good analogy to the path to fulfillment is the story of the Wizard of Oz. The goal is the starting point—to return home again with greater wisdom, greater peace of mind, and greater appreciation and control of life circumstances. The road to this goal can involve many adventures, much learning, and interesting experiences in both the inner and the outer worlds. Progress involves the discovery and resolution of tension issues, the discovery of positive states of being, and positive and constructive attitudes toward the outside world.

Times can come during relaxation practice when conceptual or emotional blocks to progress are encountered. Psychedelic sessions can help to resolve them and to open doors to new states of being. They can help a person "out of a rut" and onto a "yellow brick road".

Refinement

Refinement is a word sometimes used to describe a skillful and harmonious relationship with the outside world. An appropriate phrase could be "relaxed, effective, and dignified comportment". One of my acquaintances, a poised, elegant, and good-natured lady, once told me that she used an occasional session of "stimulated meditation" strictly to focus her continuous lifestyle practice of what she called "refining her comportment with the world". She felt that by refining and adjusting her attitudes and approaches to the world she would experience more pleasure and less stress. Her explanation was that if a person were to interact with the outside world with both her rational and her intuitive faculties of mind, she would be relating to it more completely, and with more sensitivity and effectiveness than she would if she used her rational mind alone. She says it is like using more of her mind to experience the world. Her practice involves "feeling the world right through her skin" while her rational intellect continues to participate in the process but with the advantage of additional data. She practices an extra "sixth sense" with which to become aware of profound but more subtle realities in the outside world and in relationships. She puts two and two together and finds patterns more often because of her larger perspective. She "feels" people, places, and things and new possibilities with a calmer and stronger focused attention and with what she calls "much finer precision with respect to the give-and-take moment-by-moment relationship with the world". Daily life becomes the practice of refinement. Being a conduit for positive, productive, and benevolent energy from the self to the outside world in the form of word and deed is a satisfying state of being and is the one most likely to result in positive consequences.

Of course, these sorts of explorations and practices are not restricted to women.

With refinement, even trivial tasks can become the expression of mindfulness and flow instead of the strained expression of some nervous aspect of the survival instinct. Movements of the body can become patient, relaxed, and yet precise rather than a series of jerks. We all know people with greater refinement; some are entertainers in the media. Cary Grant, Grace Kelly, and Audrey Hepburn come to mind. Such people can be used as examples to emulate. A refined image of oneself is a good addition to include in neuroplastic space, and like all such images its positive influence can echo down through all levels of the personality and into most circumstances.

After discovering a new attitude during psychedelic experience, it is possible to meditate on its possible effects on relationships to the outside world. During daily life, the new attitude can be tested for effectiveness. For instance, discovering new ways in which a soft answer can "turneth away wrath" and testing it in daily life could lead to more refined relationships. It becomes possible to debate with more objectivity despite the intensity of the mood of the debate partner.

Peace Of Mind

Another acquaintance used occasional "stimulated meditation" to help resolve enough tension issues in his inner world, in his body, and in his relationships with his outer world that he could quickly and easily let go of all of them at once and drop into the luxurious "zone of tranquility". He could enjoy the blissful feelings associated with deep relaxation along with a clear rational mind untroubled by any emotional signals associated with stress or tensions in the body. He maintains that the first key tool in developing this skill was diligent long-term practice in relaxation both with and without psychedelic stimulation, and that it has resulted in his body becoming a "mobile luxury spot". The second aspect of the task was the working through of mental tension issues that disturb tranquility by finding some kind of resolution to each of them. The third aspect was seeking and finding positive attitudes and positive points of view through meditation, psychedelic and otherwise. He considered the zone to be a "home base" that was always there, and that all he had to do was to willfully "let go of everything" in order to fall deeply into it. The memories of the resolutions of the tension issues that he found during meditation acted as "keeper bars on the horseshoe magnets" that neutralized their effects. For example, diligent meditation on finding a new way to handle a difficult relationship could neutralize future fretting sessions about it and permit a step closer to peace of mind. Meditation often results in sudden useful insights. Discarding hopeless causes and finding more reachable goals increases satisfactions and diminishes discouragements. For persistent unsolvable problems, the conviction to continue dealing with them as well as possible helps to defuse their negative influence. Sometimes the resolve to change something in the outside world is sufficient. In any case, finding keeper bar resolutions for tension issues and refining them over time is a productive activity that helps reduce ongoing tensions in the mind-body-world system. Fretting over tension issues by itself does not help to solve them.

It becomes apparent which type and amount of stress is necessary to forcefully pull one out of the zone of tranquility. That is the stress that needs to be worked on and resolved at the very moment that it is experienced in order that that the zone is once again accessible. With psychedelic stimulation, creative experiences in the form of new insights and possibilities can be a form of tension, but this feature is a satisfaction more than than a conflicting tension issue.

A time can come when just about any tension issue that can come to mind already has a resolution of some kind already worked out for it and can neutralize it. This leaves the mind free to explore neutral, positive and creative topics. These resolutions are subject to cultivation and growth as conditions, circumstances, and maturity change. This is also true with the self-chosen neuroplastic images.

After cultivating the skill of relaxing deeply, it is found that it is effortless to enter and exit from that state of being easily and quickly. Becoming active again is as easy as moving from one activity to another. Since clear situational awareness is already present, there is no wake-up period or disorientation in the process. Having the positive zone of tranquility instantly available during the day can vastly improve the quality of life, even while waiting for stoplights. Bringing more and more relaxation into the relationship with the world is part of the lifestyle of personal growth.

Dr. Grof refers to the deepest relaxation experience as the "melted ecstasy" when it is experienced during a psychedelic session. This is in contrast to what he calls the "volcanic ecstasy", or the power trip. The power trip is very healthy because it means that one has accessed the hormone that evokes the feeling of inner strength. A person can relax better when he feels strong and confident rather than when he feels weak and vulnerable.

Finding positive targets such as greater refinement and deeper relaxation within oneself gives a sense of direction to the growth process. The immediate blocks to progress are where the work needs to be done. There is no need to search for tension issues with psychedelics, they cluster into wholenesses and emerge into consciousness automatically. The more work that is done, the greater is the progress toward the positive targets. The "work" can be described as exercises in conflict resolution and the discovery of new points of view that keep them resolved. "Aha!" insights are permanent and remain effective. An ideal final target would be having peace of mind in a relaxed body that is enjoying the effects of bliss hormones while the body flows contentedly through daily life activities.

There is a saying that "some rain must fall" in everyone's life. In some people's lives, the rain can be considerable. Having cultivated the skill of using deep relaxation to escape from the anxiety and depression associated with negative circumstances can be a significant relief in a person's life. It is possible to take the plunge into the zone of tranquility for a temporary escape from the trials and tribulations of daily life. Using safe non-addicting psychedelic drugs to help to cultivate this skill is certainly a better alternative than using dangerous drugs to escape from negative feelings and then to return to circumstances that are even worse. Maintaining health and rationality can increase the likelihood of finding ways of improving or escaping from one's negative circumstances. Learning deeper acceptance and detachment from the "rain" in the human drama can also help.

Behaving in a compassionate manner toward the suffering of others can not only reduce their suffering but it can also avoid any personal guilt for ignoring it or contributing to it. Resolving guilt in order to achieve peace of mind is a real challenge; so avoiding it in the first place can be a far better approach. Abusing other people is a significant source of guilt no matter how much it might be justified. Diplomacy, consideration, and respect reduce the likelihood of confrontations and the possible accumulation of guilt, and at the same time they increase the likelihood of positive relationships.

Relaxation

The experience of deep relaxation is an absolute in that it is impossible to be any more relaxed than perfectly relaxed. It is as luxurious as anything that could be experienced at any spa or beach in the world. Being free of stress, it is healthy and rejuvenating. There are no negative emotional signals coming from a relaxed body, leaving the thought process clear, rational, and untroubled. "Reason" could be defined as a thought process processing tangible realities rather than emotional impressions. It is possible to contemplate one's life, situational problems, fantasies, and even tension issues dispassionately. A well-trained body can fall into this state instantly under most circumstances. Situational awareness is not affected. A return to activity is also instantaneous and involves no disorientation. It can be done at a stoplight. It does not interfere with an active lifestyle in the slightest. The difference is that it is possible to relax extremely deeply when so desired. It is an interesting experience to be at a movie theater, to watch extreme heartbreak or violence on the screen, and then to relax completely and view the same scenes dispassionately. Drugs and diversions are unnecessary while in this state because the peaceful luxury is totally sufficient and satisfying in itself.

The mind continues to work, but in a very clear, precise, and peaceful manner. It can be freed to ramble on its own or individual topics can be chosen for objective scrutinization. Useful insights can flow to consciousness and be recognized as such even without psychedelic stimulation. It is possible to contemplate and cultivate neuroplastic images. The neuroplastic images pertaining to peace, such as the starry sky or blissful darkness, will leave the mind-body system in a state very close to perfect peace. I believe that allowing the mind to more or less move on its own from topic to topic and back again is at least as useful overall as voluntarily using effort to stay on one topic alone.

Concentrated meditation is useful when it is needed but it is the opposite of the relaxation achieved by a mind left free to roam around topics on its own and at its own rate at any given moment. A state of being where the luxury of deep relaxation combined with an untroubled mind can relate efficiently with the outside world is a pleasant lifestyle.

Combining healthy stress-free relaxation with the laser clarity of rational thought uninfluenced by negative emotions, and with satisfying insights emerging from the intuitive mind, and with a body experiencing blissful pleasure, all combine to become a pleasant way to pass the time of day.

Faith might be defined as believing something that has never been proved, but if it acts as a "keeper bar" on a tension issue and results in a measure of tranquility and peace of mind, it is certainly is not a sin.

It takes a "well integrated" personality to achieve and maintain the tranquil state because all physical and mental tension issues have to be resolved to the extent that they can be subdued completely at least temporarily. Relaxation subdues stress hormones such as cortisol while bliss hormones such as serotonin and dopamine can still flow since they do not tense up the muscles of the body.

As with sex and anger hormones, bliss hormones can be stimulated willfully with the mind. They are felt in the skin. The skin can feel as though it is snug, tingling, and radiating such as when sunbathing, soaking in a hot tub, being massaged, or being stroked with an angora mitten. The inside of the body feels hollow because there is no no stress or tension there. A skin bathed in bliss hormones covering a stress-free hollow body with a mind blessedly at peace is about as good as it gets in this particular world. Even better might be the addition of the hormone that produces the *joie de vivre* (joy of life) emotion.

The solar plexus can feel such things as anxiety, disgust, depression, and grief. It is good to know that relaxing that area of the body can subdue those feelings. One night my daughter was out very late and she was not answering her cell phone. In the attempt to practice what I preach, I relaxed deeply and was able to subdue the feelings of extreme worry while still being entirely aware of the gravity of the situation. At another time I was able to escape at least temporarily from extreme situational depression due to a tragedy in my family. Having a safe element of natural control over emotions associated with despair in this troubles world is definitely an asset. The "inner sanctuary" is still available even under extreme stress.

Becoming more aware of hormones and the emotional experiences that they evoke can be an extremely valuable education. They can be recognized as separate realities and controlled by drugs and acts of will to a useful degree rather than being unknown invisible influences that act on their own accord to dictate our state of being and our behavior. Within the right dosage range, a psychedelic session can be mentally steered into an exploration of various hormone experiences. Some are intense, some are subtle, some are clear-cut and others are complex. There is much rich territory to be explored there. Music can be used to evoke a broad range of these experiences. There are many hormone-induced moods, many of which don't even have names. It is interesting to listen to favorite music and to notice how the moods are felt by the body and how flowing mental imagery is sometimes more appropriate than mere words to rationalize it and give it form for the sake of rational consciousness.

It is a pleasure to identify an existing subtle hormone-emotion state and then to relax it out of existence. Returning to the zone of deep relaxation and peace of mind might not be a true apotheosis, but it is a close second best. Sometimes these tension states are clearly related to current circumstances and sometimes they seem to just be there, but with practice they can often be dissolved or neutralized. A symbolic representation of this process could be the point in the movie where Dorothy steps out of her humble black-and-white house into the glorious color of Oz.

Very encouraging research is taking place testing the relatively new synthetic drug MDMA. Combined with psychotherapy, it is measurably effective in the control of posttraumatic stress disorder. I understand that it could be compared to a combination of a psychedelic drug and a euphoriant, and that it causes changes in brain functioning that are visible with MRI machines. This combination of drug effects would seem to facilitate finding positive experiences within oneself. In a video produced by the Multidisciplinary Association for Psychedelic Studies, it is stated that the hormones associated with trust, empathy, and bonding are increased while those associated with defensiveness and fear are decreased. A person seems to learn new attitudes. The science of the finer control of the hormone system will hopefully continue to make great strides.

I believe that psychedelics can make it possible for a person to first explore hormone-induced mood-attitudes and then to choose ones that he would like to make more a part of his personality. Creating an appropriate neurooplastic image for each one is of benefit because is is much easier to remember a neuroplastic mental image than to quickly change one's entire emotional and philosophic outlook into a more vague mood-attitude. Meditating on these images and mood-attitudes with and without psychedelic stimulation can make them more vivid and permanent. Such a process would help a person out of an emotional rut. For instance, a person trapped in a posttraumatic stress scenario might be able to find a new way to flow through life with greater ease and contentment. The old and the new points of view could be associated with neuroplastic images that represented them. Each of these broad abstractions could represent completely coherent clusters of individual events and feelings as perceived on the less abstract level. Rather than dealing with scattered memories and the associated feelings, they are all clustered into a single global attitude which can be solidly identified and dealt with. One or more neuroplastic images could be associated with a new attitude, which in turn could then be cultivated and put into practice. Once experienced, a new neuroplastic image can be remembered and cultivated in daily life even though it exists on a higher than normal mental level of abstraction.

Not to belabor a point too much, I believe that the clustering process and the expansion of levels of abstraction with their corresponding new insights are significant benefits of psychedelic experience. For instance, my own vivid psychedelic experience of a possible positive afterlife vastly intensified my previous one of far distant ephemeral clouds and angels. The new one was intensely experienced in my own head and it increased my daily life level of optimism and decreased my "life of quiet desperation" to significant degrees. There may be no such thing as a positive afterlife, but having a vivid conceptual experience of such a thing even one time makes it seem more possible. I have also had a vivid experience of the worst possible afterlife, but I can choose to ignore that one. At the very least I recognize them as concepts that can be experienced vividly but not necessary as representing realities anywhere else. Of course, we are free to believe whatever we wish since all of existence is a mystery. Being able to manipulate neuroplastic broad abstractions of this nature provides a greater element of control over the same hormone-emotion systems that exist at much more scattered degrees at the lower levels of abstraction. In the model that I like to use, pure mental energy can be withdrawn from one neuroplastic abstraction in the mind-brain system and channeled into another. The old abstraction stays there, but it is less often visited, of lower intensity, and perhaps involves fewer brain cells. The new image can become more vivid and visited more often. If the source of the mind is actually spirit, then it might involve fewer spirit-pixels. The concepts of brain cells and spirit-pixels are interchangeable because the source of mental activity is ultimately a mystery.

With all due respect to the miraculous complexity of the chemical-emotional hormonal process, It can at times encourage us into inappropriate or unproductive behavior. Without hormones there would be no drama in the human drama, but with them both very positive as well as very outrageous and irrational scenarios can sometimes take place. Having an element of understanding and control over the hormone system is far better than being entirely at its mercy and not even considering that it is there. For instance, if a person knew that he was temporarily under the influence of the "heartbreak" hormone, he might not be quite so convinced that his entire future life was doomed.

It is sometimes possible to mentally replay various events in one's life and to see more vividly and in more detail how outcomes might have been different if different emotional-philosophical attitudes had been taken toward them at the time. Doing so doesn't change the past but it can better prepare a person for similar events in the future. Finding smoother ways to relate to the world and to other people in various situations is one definition of "refinement".

Deep relaxation is an escape from the tensions that are built right into the human condition. Although the world has its satisfactions and pleasures, the cold hard fact is that we are frail, needy, pain-sensitive creatures having been stuck into a world that is often hostile and demanding, always uncertain, ultimately incomprehensible, while facing an unknown afterlife. We have been trapped here not by our own choosing and are forced to make the best of it regardless of circumstances. We are driven by a high-tension survival instinct filled with anxieties, fears, and flight-or-fight hormones. The stress of just being here can drive people to many forms of escape. Being stuck here is by far from the best of all possible situations. As Thoreau said, most of us live lives of quiet desperation. Deep relaxation is an escape even from even this relatively low and relatively constant sense of angst and causes a considerable brightening of the world. It can also be an ences could be classified as pertaining to such things as all-pervading spirit, creation, and causation. A person can become completely involved in one of these types of high-dose experiences much as he can in a vivid dream. Experiencing them takes a person far above the daily life level of abstraction and gives him different perspectives on the nature of existence.

The mind can create all sorts of mental material including the full range of mundane, mythical, cosmic, and religious concepts. There is plenty of inner territory to explore in there. With increasing dosage of a psychedelic it becomes possible to become more and more deeply immersed into each concept up to the point where it is almost "lived". The trick in exploring these areas is to recognize all of these points of view as concepts only and to see them rather than accept them. Points of view need to be accepted to the extent that they result in positive influences in the outside world. For instance, most people would agree that it is better to reduce someone else's suffering rather than to consider that it is his own problem. It is possible to like various points of view to varying degrees rather than to accept one as absolute. In the model that I like to use, the only absolute is that all of existence is a mystery.

Cosmic And Religious Experience

Cosmic-religious level concepts include spirit, creation, the nature of being, causation, awareness, the mind-brain boundary, the afterlife, karma, purpose, and meaning. This level of abstraction fully reveals the mystery of existence because there is no single provable answer or explanation for any one of these concepts, only assumptions. This is extremely important territory to explore especially when considering that so much of the controversy in the human drama is the result of differing cosmic assumptions and beliefs. A vivid example would be the World Trade Center disaster.

Psychedelics facilitate the exploration of cosmic assumptions because even a person who clings tightly to a particular one realizes that he is dealing only with inner mental abstractions rather than with the outside world. A very deeply religious person, for instance, could more easily explore the concept that existence unfolds strictly on the basis of natural laws.

It is tempting to add morals to the list of cosmic assumptions because there is so much controversy regarding them, but they are manmade and as such are a somewhat separate topic.

In is book *"Why Does the World Exist?"* Jim Holt reviews many of the proposed answers to cosmic concepts as suggested by famous and intelligent people throughout history and shows how none of them be validated to even the slightest extent. The ultimate reasons why they cannot be validated is because it are impossible to explain how existence could be created out of nothingness in the first place or why it happened at all. If it is assumed that God created the universe, the question becomes how God came into being. One of the more mind bending suggestions was that since God is all powerful He could create Himself. Another is that He is so pure that He does not even have to exist.

Apparently people need structure on the cosmic level so badly that they are sometimes willing to defend with their lives what ultimately amount to be nothing but assumptions. Christopher Hitchens (www. dailyhitchens.com) would call them "superstitions". Hitchens was appalled at the fact that people would seize upon and internalize cruel, violent, or even deadly superstitions out of blind faith alone even though they had no more substance than guesses made out of thin air. I am quite sure that Hitchens would call them "hot air" because these fraudulent claims are perpetrated by angry and hateful people. One example would be the actions taken by terrorists. To my knowledge, Hitchens never took the next step to point out that since all cosmic assumptions have no more substance than guesses, the entire cosmos is actually a mystery and that we should recognize all cosmic assumptions for what they really are. Of course, there is nothing harmful with positive cosmic assumptions such as the golden rule or the ten commandments.

In the unlikely event that everyone could rest comfortably in the fact that the cosmos is a mystery, it would seem that decisions could be reached much more easily and objectively than by crashing passenger jets into the World Trade Center. It would seem that the universal resolution to reduce suffering and to increase well being everywhere by taking rational steps to do so should be the prime directive of the human drama. Grappling endlessly with conflicting and abstract negative cosmic assumptions leads nowhere. Positive pragmatic practices can be tested in the material world, and such an approach should provide sufficient structure of existence for anyone.

Of course, holding any cosmic assumptions or even fantasies that successfully bring structure, peace, solace, or hope to a person would certainly not be a sin.

Spirit is obviously a mystery because there are so many assumptions regarding its being, its nature, its will, its degree of influence over daily life, and why it allows the suffering. If it were not a mystery, it would have only a single definition.

Creations is obviously a mystery. No one can explain how something came out of nothingness. As with all of the cosmic assumptions, there are many conflicting assumptions that attempt to explain it.

An illustration of the mystery of causation could involve Proteus, the hypothetical god of change. He was first conceptualized as the force that changed the sea, but over time his responsibility expanded to include the weather, the crops, and sometimes everything. If a god were responsible for all change, he would need to be aware of the location of every atom in the universe at the same time, to keep them all organized into the structures that we know, and to move them all in such a way as to cause appropriate and coherent change to take place everywhere. This process becomes extremely complex when it is working within the cells of our body and in the functioning of our brains. If it were possible to see the atomic process taking place inside of a single human cell, it would look like countless galaxies of energy-particles blending and transforming, all in exactly the right way as to magically keep the structure of the cell intact and to keep it alive. This process is truly a miracle and a mystery. A similar process takes place in our brains and presumably results in our thoughts being created. Our thoughts are immaterial virtual images and are not even composed of atoms. As such they are not even part of the material universe. In that sense, they are "the ghost in the machine" and as such closer to spirit in nature if not spirit itself. As the Dalai Lama put it, "How does the brain know what thought to think next?".

Whether Proteus is a machine running strictly on natural laws or is a spirit with awareness and intelligence or some combination of the two or something else altogether, is a mystery. Proteus himself is only hypothetical, but the function that he represents is really taking place. Some kind of unknown magic is really organizing the atoms of the universe and moving them in such a way as to cause endlessly changing configurations including those that produce the human drama. Without this clustering function taking place, the universe would be nothing but atoms in chaos like silt suspended on water. Conceptualizing change as taking place throughout the universe under the direction of a single magical force is certainly a cosmic/religious point of view. Experiencing this concept with expanded consciousness can be quite awesome, especially when realizing that modern telescopes have revealed that there are hundreds of billions of galaxies in the universe as well as that there are countless biological cells here on Earth in which countless galaxies of atoms are in constant motion. The extent to which we influence causation with our apparent free will is a mystery, but since free will *seems* to be a reality it is our responsibility to use it well.

Timothy Leary (Wikipedia) referred to this concept as the chess pieces becoming aware of the chess player and that the entire process is magic.

It would seem that the magic that can organize the flow of atoms in a single cell could also organize a world at peace. As Woody Allen put it, "The only negative thing you can say about God is that He is an underachiever".

If our here-and-now experience is conceptualized as a virtual projection of mind instead of as a product of an atomic process, then Proteus is conceptualized as purely spiritual. If Proteus is conceptualized as dreaming the atoms, then both points of view can be blended. This demonstrates how the nature of being is a mystery and how the mystery of existence can be found at all levels of abstraction. It also demonstrates how a broader abstraction can resolve conflicts at a lower level. The most abstract resolution to all cosmic conflicts is that they are all a mystery. I am quite sure that Carl Jung would call it the highest possible resolution of opposites.

A possible resolution to the mystery of causation might be on the conceptual continuum ranging from the existence of free will on the one end to the concept that God controls every atom in the universe at the other. The extent to which God controls the universe, if at all, is a mystery. At the dead center of this conceptual continuum is the point where the conflict is not even an issue. Things simply happen whether their impetus is spirit, free will, some combination of the two, or something else altogether. This is another example of how conflicts can be resolved on the cosmic level of abstraction. In some cases they can be a relief of a background mental stress.

In his book *"The Power of Intention"*, Wayne Dyer points out the notion that causation is entirely God's will. At the same time, he points out that free will seems to be a reality. He maintains that we have the choice of whether to see it one way or the other, a flexibility that has its advantages. He does not coment on the problem that if God's will controls everything, then it also controls our choice over which way to see it. In other words, the mystery of free will stays intact. The only way out of this conflict of cosmic abstractions is the broader abstraction that free will and causation are both mysteries. In other words, we cannot prove or disprove that we have free will, but it is clear that we have an *apparent* free will. As such, we are free to use it as we please without even questioning whether it is truly our own or whether is is created by spirit. In other words, we can think that we are thinking our own thoughts or that God is thinking them for us. Of course it is still our responsibility to use our apparent free will responsibly.

The "meta-concept" that all of the cosmic concepts are mysteries resolves all of the conflicts among the assumptions that claim to explain them and, as such, it can bring an element of peace of mind to anyone who is grappling with one of them. Psychedelics can facilitate this process because they expand the mind to the same level of abstraction where these concepts exist

The only thing that is provable is the consequences of living by one cosmic assumption rather than another. For example, a person who lives by the ten commandments will treat the world far differently from one who lives as a terrorist.

The nature of being is a mystery because it can legitimately be seen either as God's dream or as a material universe. In addition, it could have been created once or or creation could be a continuous process. The most basic mystery of all is how being could have emerged from nothingness.

The mind-brain boundary is a mystery because it is impossible to know how a brain, that operates with physical chemicals and atoms, could produce a three-dimensional virtual image that has no substance whatsoever. The mind is not even part of the material universe and as such is the closest thing to spirit that we can experience if not spirit itself.

With respect to the mystery of meaning and purpose, a student once asked Ramana Maharshi if it was his duty duty to join the military in order to protect his country. Ramana answered: "Your only duty is to be". In other words, we have been stuck here, not by our own choice, by unknown forces. As such, our only known reason for being here is our being here. Since all of our atoms are exchanged with the environment in a period not exceeding seven years, our existence here is a continuing miracle of complexity and by itself might be its own justification for being. Beyond this, however, we are free to choose from any number of secondary meanings and purposes as it suits us. For instance, we could become devoted to the purpose of learning as much as possible about a certain topic or perfecting a particular skill while at the same time knowing that our overall cosmic purpose is really still a mystery. We do not need to feel obligated to discover any overall meaning or purpose to existence but instead that we are free to pursue whatever captures our interest. This concept is a valuable asset for at least three reasons. One is because it frees a person from grappling with insolvable mysteries on the cosmic and religious levels. Understanding the great mystery of existence is simply not part of our job description. As such, a person is better able to focus attention on creating meaningful structures on the level of daily life. He can find and follow his own passions without doubting their authenticity. Another reason is because it makes conflict between secondary purposes unnecessary. A person is free to develop any meaningful structures that are found satisfying to him regardless of the activities that other people might be seen to choose. The third reason is that sitting peacefully doing nothing is as noble a pastime as being productive. Practicing the most pleasant and healthy state of being, luxurious deep relaxation combined with an untroubled mind, is not necessarily a shameful waste of time. Combining this state of being with an efficient relationship with the world would be the most pleasant way of flowing through this lifetime. It would certainly be better than Thoreau's "life of quiet desperation"

Structure on the everyday level has some advantages. We all need structure in this incomprehensible mystery of existence, but structure on the everyday level is concrete and useful while structure on the cosmic level can be conflicting, confusing, and in fact pure and useless guesswork. Meditating on how to refine and optimize one's relationship with the world can be far more rewarding than agonizing endlessly over how many angels can dance on the head of a pin or how creation came into being. In this way a person can enjoy the structure that he needs while at the same time being comfortable in the concept that the big picture is still a mystery.

This is certainly not to say that assumptions on the cosmic level are all bad. There are good and useful ones, such as that our cosmic purpose is to grow and to learn more about ourselves and the outside world, or that God has a plan for each one of us. These sorts of assumptions are still assumptions, but they can nevertheless bring us structure, direction. and greater peace of mind. In addition, we can choose the ones that seem truly authentic to us as individuals and to ignore any that someone else tries to impose on us.

As mentioned elsewhere, conflicts are possible at the mental cosmic level as well as at the personal level but of course they are different. An example would be the opposite concepts of determinism and free will. The question of assigning responsibility can become extremely intense at times because of this particular conflict. A conflict such as this may or may not be an issue of interest to a given individual, but if it is it could be blocking the path to tranquility. The resolution to this issue is that causation is a mystery, but actually "living" and accepting this more general concept rather than just intellectualizing it helps to further resolve any underlying tensions. A new single overall point of view can resolve tensions resulting from a conflict of separate concepts at a lower level of abstraction. "I will do what I think is right moment by moment while not being concerned with the source of my decisions" can replace the conflict between "what will be will be so I am helpless and not responsible" and "I am totally responsible for everything that happens to me and everything that I do in my lifetime". I am guessing that resolutions of this nature could be correlated with neuroplasticity where a new neural network in the brain is energized. By analogy, mental energy can flow around the new city bypass rather than through the traffic in the city itself and be that much closer to tranquility.

It can be imagined how the resolution of a somewhat similar cosmic conflict might make it unnecessary for a person to take high risks in order to prove to himself whether fate is on his side or not. He would no longer need to either trust or to defy the hypothetical cosmic/mythical "personal protector" within his cosmic conceptual realm. Instead he could relax, let come what may, and to deal with his fate as it actually unfolds as well as possible. He would no longer have to hurtle through space on a motorcycle or bet the entire farm in order to find out if the powers that be will really protect him or not. Instead, he could see the opposing concepts of doubt and trust existing only in his own mind, see them as equal and opposite forces, and as such see the whole issue as a combination of balanced forces that could be resolved and set aside. There is no way for anyone to know what fate has in store for us, so the best answer is to take it as it comes and deal with it the best way possible rather than to tempt or defy it. Any future leanings toward one or the other of the lower level abstractions would hopefully evoke the memory of the resolution and nullify any conflict that might try to get started.

The religious experiences are the most abstract, the highest, and the most exalted of all of the concepts. There are no words to describe their grandeur. The emotions felt while experiencing them include those of breathtaking awe and wonder. The mind becomes capable of conceptualizing and becoming fully immersed in such abstractions as pure all-pervading space and all-pervading spirit. It can also conceptualize the astounding complexity of the countless galaxies of atoms that need to be organized, either by spirit or otherwise, in order to organize our bodies and our here-and-now environment, and then to be constantly rearranged in order to generate endless change taking place everywhere. Also to be recognized is the unity of the body, the mind, and all-pervading space and/or spirit. One senses absolute cosmic purity and an overwhelming approval of existence in all of its wholeness. When a person who has experienced this state and claims to be God, he is really saying that he has convincingly experienced the broad mental abstraction that everything is God.

There is substantial literature in this area contributed by people of many cultures who have had the same sorts of experiences with and without psychedelic drugs.

Although the religious experience is overwhelmingly convincing, there is no way to prove that it actually reflects reality. Modern MRI research has supposedly revealed a "God spot" in the brain that is activated during religious experience. This can be researched on the Internet. It does not prove that the religious experience is nothing but an inner subjective experience, however, because it is always possible that God activates that part of the brain Himself during those experiences or even that all of reality is actually His dream. In any case, it is an obvious fact that something holds this universe together and keeps changing its structure.

The mystery of existence remains fully intact in spite of the religious experience. In my own personal experience, God (or what might only be my concept of God) is not offended by being considered as mysterious, and doing so does not cause any conflict in the mental realm of cosmic concepts.

I am quite sure that anyone who chooses to explore the cosmic regions of the psychedelic experience will eventually end up concluding that even though existence is miraculous and magnificent, it is nevertheless absolutely mysterious. I once asked my "hypothetical inner spiritual teacher" (no offense intended, Lord) if He were really God or just my imagination. What came back was the answer "You don't know, do you?" To me, that says it all. Of course, everyone is free to reach their own conclusions regarding matters of spirit. I personally consider that paying homage to the miraculous and majestic quality of existence, however it came into being, is a form of worship.

There are two general ways to define existence: the materialistic and the spiritualistic. Since all of existence is a mystery, there is no sense agonizing too much over the degree to which either one is "accurate" or even if there is yet another answer that is beyond our comprehension. In fact, there is little reason to agonize over anything that is an unsolvable mystery. Clearly, the here-and-now moment is all that exists, and from the materialistic viewpoint it is made entirely of atoms arranged in space. What it is that keeps these atoms organized is a mystery, so I would just as soon call it "magic" to avoid conflicts between the spiritualistic and the materialistic definitions of causation. A broader abstraction of this nature smooths out the flow of mental energy throughout the mental cosmic abstractions at lower levels, neutralizes conflicts between the various "cosmic assumptions", and permits another step forward toward peace of mind.

The Spiritual Definition

The most clear-cut spiritual perspective is that an all-pervading God controls the position of every atom in the universe at every single moment. The whole process is His including the smallest wisp of every human thought. A more complex perspective is that He controls specific parts of it on occasion but leaves the rest to the natural laws that He has already created and to the free will that He permits us to exercise. These points of view can become very vivid and experienced very deeply during high-dose psychedelic sessions.

Many other assumptions need to be made if the spiritual definition of existence is assumed: Why and how did God create the universe? What is its purpose? Why are we here? What system of morals does He want us to live by? Do our thoughts emerge from a material brain or does He create them? Does He listen to prayers? Do rituals influence future events? Why does He let so many terrible things happen? Did He give us free will? Is evolution a reality? Many assumed answers have been proposed regarding these sorts of questions and others like them throughout history, but none of them can be proved or disproved to even the slightest extent. It is possible to experience and contemplate these sorts of questions and proposed answers during a high-dose psychedelic experience and it is possible to see how the answers can conflict with one another. Considering how much effort that highly intelligent people have put into finding answers in these areas, it is clear that there is a strong human need for structure in them. I am convinced that sufficient exploration of these areas will eventually convince anyone that the answer is that there is no answer. We are trapped in a "philosophical void" in this regard, but recognizing the miraculous and the magnificent aspects of existence and its complexity on the atomic level helps to compensate for our inability to comprehend or to know its source, nature, or purpose. Until some form of proof comes to light, if ever, the most authentic definition of existence would be that it is a fantastic mystery. Appreciation of its scope and miraculous and magnificent nature makes up for not having answers to it.

Appreciating this awesome reality is, to me, a form of worship.

The model that I like to use is that it is possible to hold beliefs while at the same time accepting that ultimately they are improvable. Working with psychedelics seems to make it more clear that it is possible to hold one point of view at one time and then another at another time while at the same time being aware of both of them and while not experiencing conflict in choosing the one or the other to consider at any given moment. Different structures can be used to explain the same realities, an example being the wave theory and the particle theory of light or the liberal and the conservative definitions of politics.

The biblical story of the Tower of Babel suggested that people could not communicate because of differences in language, but in effect we also have a great deal of trouble communicating with each other because of different believed answers regarding the great mystery of existence. One only needs to listen to politicians or people from different religions in the same culture argue to get a glimpse of this fact. Some of the different assumptive points of view might be vividly experienced during a high dose experience, but a time can come when it appears as though they are all incomplete but necessary methods to give structure to something that is ultimately impossible to define with certainty.

The only really solid footholds that we have in this existence are the absolutely reliable natural laws and the more general cause-effect relationships that result from the interactions between them. Our mission in life seems to be to learn these relationships insofar as possible and to use them productively.

As the spiritualistic Deepak Chopra puts it, existence is God's dream, we are dreamers within His dream, and we project the dream out into what appears to be an outside world. Existence is a unity in the sense that all of it is God's single universal dream. The religious experiences can be extremely beautiful:

> Suspended in the bliss of Nirvana
> Touched by a tentative thought
> Then merged gain with the infinite sea
> Brought home, again, to Thee

With perfect precision and tiny divisions
This delicate filigree
With lines so fine they start to combine
With celestial purity

The Materialistic Definition

Probably the most popular materialistic point of view regarding creation would be the big bang theory. In this case, all of the matter, energy, space, and time in the universe somehow exploded out of nothingness. Existence is made entirely of atoms that move and combine strictly according to natural laws. With an assumed intelligent spirit out of the picture, natural laws by themselves somehow continue to move the atoms of existence in such a way as to produce everything in the universe. The discovery of the Higgs-Boson particle might explain how mass has gravity, but it will shed little light on the mystery of how atoms are kept in continual motion to produce the human drama.

One implication to this point of view is that destiny is predetermined since natural laws are absolutely fixed in their expression and no other influences are present. Another implication is that free will is an illusion since the atoms in our brains are processing information strictly according to natural laws. I am sure that Einstein had a great respect for natural laws, and he said that he did not like the idea that God played dice with the universe, but I am not sure of the degree to which he considered God to be responsible for causation. But even if he thought that God did not contribute at all to causation and that material laws ruled the universe, it would seem that he would have to concede that the universe had to come from somewhere.

One rather exotic way to structure this particular concept would be to assume that the entire history of the universe is stored in memory somehow. As the current moment moves through it, our experience is generated. Some have suggested that the universe is a very long "tape loop" that plays over and over.

The conflict between the concepts of free will and determinism is resolved by recognizing that the answer is a mystery. Once that it done, the conflict can be ignored and it is possible to relax and simply do what seems to be right moment by moment. What seems to be right is based on our entire past experience, so the current assumptions that are made can be trusted to be at least as productive as they had been in the past.

If this super-complex energy process is not seen as unfolding exclusively by itself but instead by some percentage of intelligent influence, then a gradation from a materialistic to a spiritualistic points of view can become apparent. The assumed percentage of intelligent influence of causation becomes the big question. It could be that all causation is the result of a spiritual prime mover or it could be the result of all natural laws or some combination of the two or something else we cannot even conceptualize. Anyone who believes in the effectiveness of prayer believes that there is a degree of flexibility in the flow of destiny.

In any case, the unfolding universe is a monumental process of data management. Without the mysterious cosmic "organizing principle" at work, the universe would be atoms in chaos.

An overall perspective could be that it is "magic" that moves the atoms of existence. It can be defined as acting on along a continuum ranging from the materialistic on the one end to the spiritualistic on the other end. We can choose any point on this spectrum as an answer to the mystery of causation and move around on it as we wish or as circumstances dictate. We can also choose the center point and ignore the entire conceptual polarity and conclude that what is simply is what is.

I think that this flexibility of thought can reduce a lot of tension on the mental level of cosmic abstractions and can permit another step forward toward peace of mind. To be completely peaceful, it is necessary to be able to "let things be" as they are.

In other words, causation can be conceptualized as a mystery, and relaxing in a mystery is less stressful than agonizing over an unsolvable conflict.

If the mysterious energy that unfolds the destiny of the universe were to shut off, what would be left would be absolutely pure infinite and eternal space with no energy-atoms present. This image can be conceptualized mentally and cultivated in neuroplastic space as a symbol of perfect peace and purity if so desired:

> The endless vastness of space
> A silent witness is seeing
> No disturbance anyplace
> Only perfect Being

The cosmic concept of pure empty space involves perfect peace of mind and a perfectly relaxed body. Sri Aurobindo (www.aurobindo.net) referred to this particular concept as being so pure that it does not even a ripple in it in order to exist. On the other hand, the cosmic concept of a single atom suspended and stationary in pure and empty space requires maximum focussed concentration. Both of these most abstract neuroplastic images lead to relaxation of the body, focussed serenity, and mental and physical health. As such are worthy of cultivation.

Everything in our material existence is permeated through and through with a single volume of invisible space. Vibrating "principles" move through this single volume of space thus creating what appears to us as atoms moving along their paths. The "principles" move through space like laser images move through mist without disturbing the position of the droplets in the least. Space itself is imperturbable except for the presence or the absence of vibrating energy-atoms. Seeing points of view such as this can come as a surprise during psychedelic experience and, as always, are a mystery.

Ambiguity Tolerance

I believe that accepting the fact that existence and spirit are complete mysteries and that we mere mortals are simply not privileged to know the answers is the one of the most comfortable approaches to take if one chooses to explore the cosmic and religious levels of the psychedelic experience. It is possible to explore and become involved with any of the assumed answers without running into significant conflicts except in areas where our own personal assumptions have reached the level of beliefs. At those points our individual beliefs will likely be seen as being only one of many different possibilities but nevertheless the ones we have chosen to live by. Examples would be all of the different definitions of the afterlife, all of the different guesses regarding God's motives and agenda, the purpose of existence, and the proper system of morals to live by. The assumption that everything is a mystery neutralizes all of the conflicts, and yet we are still free to abide by the assumptions that seem most plausible and authentic to us and the ones that we are most comfortable to live by. No doubt our choices are based mostly on our own personal real-life experiences, and they change very little even after multiple high doses psychedelic experiences and even then still by choice. Each of us only sees a portion of the world, so we naturally draw our conclusions on the basis of what we have seen. Psychedelics do not brainwash a person into a specific set of values, but they provide a great deal of new flexibility of perspective. When we do run into conflicts at the cosmic level of abstraction, the trapdoor concept that everything is a mystery is always available. It is on a higher level of abstraction and as such it transcends all of the conflicts on the lower levels of abstraction. One "looks down" on all of the conflicts on all the lower levels.

Carl Jung assumed that all emotional conflicts have their roots on this level of abstraction. If this is the case and if psychedelic experience can help to resolve them, the process should be very therapeutic. I believe that this is indeed the case. Perhaps Mother Theresa would not have had to endure her crisis of faith if she had accepted the fact that it is ultimately impossible to prove or to disprove the existence of a mysterious God.

The great religions of the world claim to know some of the cosmic answers to existence, but since none of these answers can be proved or disproved, their claims have yet to be validated. Of course, many of the assumed answers are eminently useful, such as those pertaining to moral behavior.

The religious experience can not only sometimes be reached with a high dose of a psychedelic drug, it can also be remembered and approached later with much lower doses and even in normal daily consciousness. It is basically a single concept: that existence is an absolutely mysterious unity of being composed of all-pervading space, spirit, or some combination of the two, and that everything and each of us is part of it. Actually we are trapped inside of it and cannot establish an external frame of reference to it. This explains the koan that a finger cannot point to itself. In addition, our personal awareness is a unity and so is the field of experience that we are aware of: the "trinity" of mind, body, and outside world.

> If a scientist, made of dough
> Took a ruler made of dough
> And measured objects made of dough
> What exactly would he know?

At least he could investigate the cause-effect relationships that exist within the dough and he could strive to mold it into the most rewarding configurations possible.

A resolution to the opposites of the physical and the spiritual definitions of existence could start with the concept that we actually live only in our minds, and that our mental experience is the only provable reality. However the word "mind" implies the output of a physical brain, so if there really is no physical brain because the entire physical world is all in our mind, then another word is needed to take the place of "mind". The word "experience" does so. We experience (verb) nothing but our own experience (noun) and we know that it really exists. This is as far as we can go and remain logically authentic. Any other assumptions regarding its source or its composition or its purpose go beyond the data. As Alan Watts put it: "This is it and this is all there is".

The source of our experience is as mysterious as the "magic" that organizes the atoms of the universe into the structures that we know.

It is also possible to look for cause-effect-relationships within what we normally consider to be mental experience itself. For instance, the cultivation of positive neuroplastic images is found to be truly effective. Questions regarding the influence of free will on the overall process, if there is any, can be ignored because even those questions are part of the experience. So we can go ahead and look for cause-effect-relationships all we want because even wanting to do so is part of the experience. We are literally a part of our here-and-now immediate moment-by-moment experience whatever it is and whether we are thinking or acting or both. Experience itself is a oneness and as such transcends the opposites of spirit and matter, which in turn are concepts that are part of that experience. Experience itself is everything.

On the one hand, the concept that existence is a mystery is a philosophical void, but it has two significant advantages. One is that it resolves all conflicts between assumptions regarding the nature if existence, some of which can lead to considerable conflict both within oneself an between people. On the other hand is that one is not trapped by any given assumptions and is free to find and to live by the ones that prove to be the most productive and good.

Neuroplastic Influence

Mentioned earlier was the fact that MRI research has revealed that religious monks who meditate long on compassion for the human condition activate specific areas of their brains. I have discovered that something similar takes place when selected concept-images are contemplated and cultivated both during psychedelic experience and daily life, but I really have no knowledge of any corresponding neuroplastic changes in the brain. In any case, I like to refer to them as neuroplastic images for the sake of simplicity. With repetition and meditation these concept-attitude-images can become quite vivid and real mentally, and they can influence daily life to a surprising extent. Meditation can be used to select the most pleasant and the most useful images to cultivate in neuroplastic space. Just as memory-joggers can remind us of names or words, neuroplastic images can remind us of entire experiences including attitudes and states of being. With enough cultivation, they can even become sources of diversion during meditation periods. As an example, I would like to describe the most spectacular neuroplastic concept-image that I have ever experienced.

About thirty years ago I had a high dose LSD experience in which I found myself identifying with a woman wandering lost in a blizzard. I was carrying my baby who had already died of the cold. I don't pretend to know where these little "vignettes" come from in the mind-brain, but they are always spontaneous, detailed, and realistic, and they reveal unusual circumstances as seen through another person's eyes. I consider them as being produced by the intuitive mind in order to communicate insights in dramatic form. They are not always negative in quality; they can also be quite positive. In this story, I finally sat down in the snow to accept death. I felt that at least I had my faith in God and in heaven, but when I tipped my head forward and closed my eyes, all I could see was a preposterous inner cartoonland. My life had been a complete absurd farce. Between the biting cold on the outside and the cartoonland on the inside, the only relief in sight seemed to be the peaceful darkness of approaching death.

When the peaceful darkness flowed over me, I surrendered to it completely. Death is the ultimate act of letting go. However, when a person lets go to such a high degree while still alive in the real world, a cascade of bliss hormones can take place due to the extremely deep relaxation. This can make death seem like an extremely positive experience. It was like being a disembodied mind liberated of all earthly cares suspended in a domain of perfect peace, bliss, and purity. It is easy to surrender to something positive. My old concept of death involved dead bodies moldering underground in scary cemeteries at night with werewolves howling at the moon. The new one was considerably better. Even though it might have been nothing more than a fraudulent brainwashing by a chemical, it was a good one. It became the basis of a new neuroplastic image that I still meditate upon. Fortunately, you don't have to be dead to enjoy some deep level of this particular experience.

I noticed in the days that followed my "positive death experience" that my anxiety level associated with my survival instinct was much reduced. The "life of quiet desperation" that Thoreau referred to diminished significantly and life became much brighter. I was surprised to discover how much of daily life actually dealt with the survival and well-being concerns and in one way or another. Examples would be competition in the workplace, efforts to maintain health, ambition, greed, and crime. Even reading the newspaper is a form of vigilance toward possible threats. Death is such a pervasive overarching reality in daily life that a positive attitude toward it makes a big difference in attitude and mood.

Much more recently my doctor called and told me that I had cancer. I was instantly fully prepared for the heavy hit of high anxiety in my solar plexus, but absolutely nothing happened. The information went through my mind like a laser image through mist. The first thought that sprung to mind was the "neuroplastic positive image" of death. This demonstrates, at least for me, the significant power of neuroplastic images. This one was stronger than my survival instinct, and no doubt the survival instinct is deeply imbedded in our biology. Later, after surgery, I was pronounced cancer free. I will not go so far as to say that I was disappointed, but I also took this news in a relatively matter-of-fact manner.

If it were somehow possible to make this experience available to terminally ill people, it would vastly reduce their anxiety. The same would be true for their close friends and relatives. "Going to a better place" could become more of a believable possibility even if it is only a concept stimulated by a chemical. However, since the afterlife is a mystery, it could actually be true. There is always hope. Perhaps there will someday be a safe drug that promotes this or similar experiences. The psychedelic experience is somewhat unpredictable, so there is no guarantee that it would do so. At the same time, it might be possible for a terminally ill person, or anyone else for that matter, to meditate upon and cultivate a neuroplastic image of letting the body and the mind melt into peaceful blissful darkness. Some people might prefer light or some other neuroplastic image, but bliss is bliss regardless of the associated image. In my own case, I use that image among others during meditation practice in order to reach the deepest possible state of relaxation and contentment, and I hold out hope that death will prove to be as positive as that.

Deep relaxation is healthy as well as pleasant because there is no stress. The body gets a chance to heal itself and the immune system gets a chance to strengthen itself.

I still look both ways before I cross the street because I still know that the afterlife is a mystery and because the practical side of my survival instinct is still fully intact. I can still slam on the brakes as fast as anyone.

Another neuroplastic image that I have rather firmly cultivated in my mind is the "mature good-natured objective diplomat". I can meditate on its qualities even while it is smoothing my relationships with and between other people. Another is the "relaxed housekeeper" who pleasantly flows through daily mundane chores and obligations rather than hating them the way that I used to. Another is a giant ultramodern luxury cruise liner standing absolutely stationary and suspended in the crystalline waters of a beautiful lagoon. Stillness of the body helps to maintain the serene state. The little waves that lap against the side of the ship can represent the daily concerns that come to mind, and they will have no negative effect. A deeply relaxed person feels suspended because he lets all of his weight down on whatever is supporting him; he has no inclination to jump up and do something. One with many interesting aspects is the empty suit of shining armor that can move around like an ordinary person. It represents honor, the ability to defend oneself against the slings and arrows of outrageous fortune, and the care not to behave in such a way as to accumulate internal tension issues. For instance, abusing someone causes guilt,and guilt leads to damage and conflict in the self image which in turn leads to depression. Emptiness in this regard is to be preferred. These sorts of images and others like them jump to mind under appropriate circumstances in daily life and influence one's current attitude and state of being.

Neuroplastic images of different sorts can be associated with a variety of different states of being and their corresponding attitudes. These images represent individual clustered organizations of points of view, states of the body, and attitudes towards oneself, the outer world, and the cosmos. They can be cultivated and improved upon over time and their influence can be observed and felt in daily life.

I believe that self-chosen positive neuroplastic images of this nature can act not only to provide elements of objective control over any existing negative ones, but also to act as "guiding lights" through the made of life.

Managing Bad Trips

The psychedelic experience usually tends to be expansive and positive, but there is always the the possibility of a "bad trip" at times. For this reason, it is good to be ready to handle one if it should start to take place. It helps to remember rationally that psychedelics can cause a vivid amplification of any number of philosophic points of view combined with their corresponding emotions, and that they can be negative as well as positive. A person should see himself as exploring various concepts on an abstract level of mental experience rather than as viewing what might sometimes appear to be realities.

I am sure that the best way to handle a bid trip is to relax insofar as possible and to let the experience exhaust itself rather than to fight it or run from it. As with all cosmic and religious concepts, it helps to remember that one is experiencing a vivid philosophical and emotional identification with a mental concept, not necessarily with an actual reality. Finding the heart of one of these experiences can be a satisfying relief and even educational.

The unfortunate fact is that there is plenty of negativity in the human drama, so unavoidable meditation on how to handle and solve various everyday problems can be expected at times. This is not really not too much of a problem with low to moderate doses of a psychedelic drug because the expanded rational mind and the sensitive intuitive mind can work together very effectively to find legitimate answers to existing everyday situations. This kind of meditation can actually be very satisfying and profitable.

I believe that the really bad trip (the "bummer") is almost always due to an inexperienced person taking too high a dose under poor circumstances. The higher dose causes the experience to deal with abstract "cosmic" issues rather than daily life issues, so it would be helpful if anyone acting as ground control were familiar with this level of abstraction. I also believe that these bad experiences will take place at the beginning of the trip because it can look as though something extremely dangerous is coming from nowhere and overwhelming the mind. Therefore, it would be a good practice to gain experience with lower doses under positive circumstances if one makes the choice to dabble with psychedelics at all. If an experienced person should run into a bad trip, he would be far more able to maintain the rational perspective and flow through it while it happened. He would know that it would pass. These sorts of trips can be quite educational both in terms of psychology itself and in terms of facing, dealing with, and accepting real negative aspects in the human drama that can and do reflect themselves in one's personal life drama.

From a strictly rational and objective viewpoint, the human condition has a significant downside, so sometimes parts of psychedelic trips can be a little grim. Denying the negative aspects of the human condition would be self-delusion and exploring them would expand a person's breadth of human knowledge, his compassion for others, and his ability to face, accept, and endure unpleasant facts in daily life.

We find ourselves having been inserted here, not by our own choice, into these frail, needy, pain-sensitive human bodies living in a world that is often hostile and demanding, always uncertain, and ultimately incomprehensible. We know that tragedy can strike at any moment. The maze of life can be quite challenging, overwhelming, and bewildering at times.

We don't know how we got here, why we are here, or how or why this place exists at all. We know that we will eventually leave it and we can only guess what comes afterwards. The religious monks who change the neuroplastic configuration of their brains through meditation on compassion toward the human drama certainly have plenty to work with.

The best we can hope for in this fleeting lifetime is an average state of reasonably positive well-being and as harmonious a relationship with the outside world as possible. We can strive and do what is necessary to make progress toward these goals. Psychedelic experience can help by providing intuitive sensitivity and broader perspectives to the process.

Humphrey Osmond came up with a poem that is rather famous in the psychedelic world:

> To fathom Hell or soar angelic
> Just take a pinch of psychedelic

Another approach is to encourage the experience "do its worst". Either it will eventually die out or the "heart" of it will be found. I remember in my own case that the heart of one bad trip was symbolized by the rather exotic symbol of a bush being blown by the wind. The wind whipped the bush into the shape of a human face expressing agony. I could see that it represented the fact that we are all trapped and rooted here, not in a bush but in the here-and-now moment regardless of what it might contain. In addition, there are people all around the world every day who are trapped in constant extreme negative circumstances. Finding a resolution to this extremely tragic cosmic fact without being outraged, frightened, or repulsed by it took quite a bit of work on both the mundane and the cosmic levels of abstraction. I saw the entire human race as treading water struggling to stay afloat and many people being unable to do so and going under. Eventually everyone goes under. From the spiritualistic point of view, I had to accept that God lets terrible things happen. From the materialistic point of view, I had to accept that terrible things were programmed into a predetermined destiny driven by fixed natural laws and that we are stuck in a cosmic storybook that has some very grizzly chapters. Compassion for the suffering became the dominant attitude toward this unfortunate part of reality instead of the conflicting attempts to fix the blame for it. Contemplating suffering is certainly a bad trip.

Resolving to make efforts to reduce my own suffering and that of the people I encounter in daily life to the extent possible was a partial solution to this particular tension issue in my case. Reducing suffering is a higher moral activity than is ignoring it, fretting about it, or contributing to it. Opportunities to reduce various forms of suffering, mild or extreme, can occur continuously in everyday life. Another part of the solution was the resolution to contribute to the upside of the human drama insofar as possible by treating people with goodwill and respect. Psychologically this combination is a win-win situation because negativity is reduced in both the inner and the outer worlds. If a person is doing what he can to increase the upside and decrease the downside in his own little corner of the world, he knows that at least he is moving some things into positive directions and he can feel good about it.

The broad cosmic assumption that finally emerged that significantly helped to resolve the problem of suffering was the "yin-yang" transcendental concept that in order for existence to exist at all, the forces of creation and the forces of destruction need to be in balance. Although the flow of destiny can be seen as the continual rearrangement of atoms, it can also be seen as atoms being arranged in creative and destructive fashions. From this point of view, the creative forces and the destructive forces need to be equal since they are both part of the same process. If the forces of creation dominated, eventually everything would be created and change would cease. If the destructive forces dominated, eventually the universe would be atoms in chaos. The yin-yang principle seems to be true in the cosmos with respect to the birth and death of stars, and it seems true here on Earth where all life eventually dies and gets recycled through the topsoil. The super-complex creation of life on Earth, as seen from the perspective of the "magical" forces that organize the atoms that make up all of existence, might need a compensating "disorganizing" aspect that could ultimately account for the suffering in the human drama. Even the process of our aging contains creative and destructive aspects. Accurate or not, this particular balancing concept helped to resolve my mental tension on the cosmic level of mental abstraction and to permit another step toward peace of mind. Instead of feeling outrage toward ruthless dictators who massacre their own citizens in the streets, such suffering could be explained and accepted in a more neutral fashion as a necessary condition in order for the big picture to exist at all. It is not too far from the God-Devil concept except that it assumes that causation is in fact the rearrangement of atoms. It is an authentic resolution since the troubling negative emotions that would exist otherwise serve no purpose anyway. What is is what is warts and all and the best we can do is to try to make it better.

A way to handle this fact of reality would be to channel the inevitable forces of destruction into ways that minimize the suffering that can be associated with them. Many efforts have already been made in this direction. Medical science is an example as are the attempts to create equitable and benevolent political and economic systems within countries. We all still age and die, but the process has made much more tolerable with medicines, artificial joints, and other procedures. Reestablishing mental hospitals would ease the suffering of the homeless. Democratic forms of government allow peaceful change whereas dictatorships often involve massacre in the streets. Family planning involves a degree of sacrifice, but it would clearly involve less suffering than poverty, overcrowding, or battles for territory or resources. Adjusting the definition of work and the appropriate compensation for it could reduce the suffering associated with technological unemployment and unemployment due to other reasons. If a person were compensated for "productive potential" through education as well as for actual production, he would be motivated to remain educated for possible later contributions to society while not actually being productive at the time. He would be motivated to advance his education and to remain well-rounded instead of giving up and living under a bridge. If society and technology could somehow guarantee a reasonable basic subsistence living for people for whom homelessness would be the only alternative, perhaps the extent of desperate greedy behavior to assure personal survival at high secure levels would be reduced and inequities in the financial system would be fewer. Job failure would not be as threatening, so stepping on other people's fingers would not be as necessary. Using technology to recycle and to utilize renewable energy resources reduces shortages of non-renewable natural resources and the suffering that results from them. Methods of achieving greater relaxation and peace of mind, such as those suggested here and elsewhere, could reduce the tensions associated with having been stuck into this sometimes-hostile, always uncertain, and ultimately incomprehensible world while at the same time being programmed with intense survival emotions. An ideal pie-in-the-sky situation would be where all of the inevitable forces of destruction could be channeled into areas of minimal suffering.

As computers drive more and more of the machines that provide our goods and services, the worldwide historical stressful struggle for survival and security should diminish. More satisfying and fulfilling pastimes and activities for humanity could hopefully be found as the machines continued to do their work. We would not have to spend so much time hunting for food in the jungle or the modern equivalent thereof. It seems that the marketplace and the various political systems should adjust naturally and hopefully painlessly to this new and growing blessing in the history of mankind.

The top level of mental abstraction regarding the nature of existence is pure, infinite, eternal, all-pervading space. Next down is all-pervading space shared with all-pervading spirit. Next down is the creation of atoms, either emerging or having emerged from space or from spirit or from both. Next down is the magical process of the continuous arrangement and rearrangement of the atoms that make up the structures that we know such as suns, planets, and individual human cells. Next down is the yin-yang concept where the unfolding process of existence at the atomic level is conceptually divided into the two equal forces of creation and destruction in all of their complexity. The destructive forces include wear and damage, both of which can involve suffering. The next level down is where a person thinks about events, patterns, and influences in his daily life. The lowest level of abstraction is the actual here-and-now involvement in the flow of events that make up daily life.

The top six levels of abstraction are strictly mental, so there is plenty to explore in those regions. For instance, contemplating the top level can lead to deeper peace of mind and tranquility. Contemplating the second and third levels can stimulate a deeper appreciation for the miracle and the mystery of creation emerging from nothingness. Contemplating the fourth level down can stimulate an appreciation of such magic as how the atoms making up a single human cell can extract exactly the right atoms from the bloodstream, process them in exactly the right way to keep the cell alive, and then to release them back into the bloodstream in transformed configurations. This process would be equivalent to galaxies merging and intermingling. Contemplating the fifth level down can help to explain the existence and nature of suffering. Everything that is created including living beings, structures, and empires must eventually be changed or destroyed in one way or another. Purposefully engineering the most peaceful possible change under all possible circumstances would be desirable. Contemplating the daily life level on the sixth mental level can help us to figure out ways to maximize the likelihood of well-being and to minimize the many various forms of discontent which exist on the seventh level, the level of the experience of daily life.

Viewing existence from a transcendental viewpoint such as its miraculous quality can have a psychological benefit. The trivial, absurd, and other unpleasant aspects of existence can become more easily tolerated and can be replaced with a more tension-free mental acceptance and appreciation of them. The human drama and one's own personal drama can be viewed from a more objective and a less emotional perspective.

Assuming that it is true that psychedelics can lead to greater psychological satisfaction and fulfillment, they would represent a constructive force in society. To the extent that they can compensate for the destructive forces of anxiety, depression, hostility, confusion, and greed in society, their influence will have plenty of room to grow.

Once I accepted the transcendental "yin-yang" assumption as a possibility to explain suffering, my bad trip lost steam and moved on to a much more positive topic: if the constructive and the destructive forces of the cosmos were to conceptually cancel each other out completely, what would be left would be a concept of pure, empty, tension-free peaceful, infinite, and eternal space which in turn equates to perfect peace of mind. Peace of mind in turn equates to a relaxed body experiencing bliss hormones and a positive state of being in the here-and-now moment. This is an example of how conflicts at even the cosmic level of abstraction can be resolved with even broader concepts just as is the case in the mythical and everyday levels of abstraction.

The paranoid experience is one where the threats in existence are conceptualized as conspiratorial or supernatural or both. Even in normal daily consciousness it is not too hard to conceptualize that a hypothetical "god of war" or a collusion of hawkish conspirators influenced the rush to war with Iraq. On the cosmic level of psychedelic experience such hypothetical influences can appear much more vivid, personal, and real due to the clustering effects of stimulated intuitive thought. In any case, the most effective way to deal with these experiences is the same as with all other "bad trips": let them do their worst. The mind actually seems to desire to finally face the heart of a negative experience and to get it over with and to neutralize it. During psychedelic experience, the real-world reality of the perceived threat is not the main issue. The issue is to face it squarely in the mental world regardless of its corresponding degree of reality in the material world. The evaluation of the objective reality of the threat in the material world can be postponed until the emotional amplifications stimulated by the psychedelic drug are over.

It is possible to handle a bad trip by finding its heart, surrendering to it, and going through it. It can be a significant learning experience. As one of my clients put it: "Once you have been eaten by one mouth, you have been eaten by all of them". Revisiting the same areas in the future can be on a much more objective level and can actually be doorways to new areas of exploration. For instance, it can become possible to investigate practical ways to reduce the downside of the human drama and to contribute to its upside even within one's little corner of the world.

If a person having a bad trip recognized that he was actually in a temporary hormonal/chemical state of being, he might also have the courage to take the opportunity of exploring it to some extent while it lasted. There is a great deal to learn about how hormones can prejudice our perceptions.

Sometimes it might take more than one psychedelic session and perhaps some daily meditation in order to find the heart of a tension issue. The cosmos is a big place.

If ground control is present, as it should be during high dose sessions, and if it can offer reassurances of current safety, encourage endurance and surrender, and at the same time to promote the rational perspective, so much the better.

Since existence is uncertain, one never knows how vigilant and cautious to be. What appears to be too much fear, anxiety, and caution might at times be just enough, but during a psychedelic session in good surroundings with a trusted and experienced companion, negative experience can be revealed as strictly irrational, not real, and something that can be dealt with since it is only chemically-induced mental imagination and hormone reactions. It is possible to recognize bad trips for what they are and to let them go right on by.

Letting bad trips go right on by is a form of good practice for letting negative situations in daily life go right on by. Challenges can be faced and dealt with on a more objective level and with less frantic anxiety. To put it poetically, once a person has faced the core of Hell, all other threats pale in significance. Endurance and patience can be practiced as useful forms of strength to deal with the downside of the human drama.

> When the badness of Hell
> Meets the goodness of Heaven
> In the center of cosmic space
> They may start to entwine
> Or even combine
> In a kind of a cosmic embrace

As long as we have been stuck here on Earth anyway, we might as well look for ways to make our short stay here as comfortable as reasonably possible. If resolving conflicts at the cosmic level of abstraction helps to do so, so much the better. Otherwise we might as well leave them alone and stick with lower doses of psychedelic drugs for the sake of self-exploration, relaxation, or diversion or to abandon them altogether. Abandoning psychedelic drugs altogether is hardly a problem; I did so for thirty years with no problems whatsoever.

Summary

Lines from a few classic songs suggest productive belief-attitudes (faiths) that can be taken toward our earthly situation that will facilitate peace of mind.

"I am just a weary pilgrim, plodding through this world of sin," suggests attitudes of acceptance, endurance, and determination in the face of difficulties in an unknown fate. To the extent that a person can accept the fact that he has been temporarily stuck here in a human body that is frail, needy, and pain-sensitive while living in a world that is sometimes hostile and demanding, always uncertain, and ultimately incomprehensible, he can endure the more negative circumstances of life more easily and thereby enjoy deeper peace of mind. At the same time he is still free to enjoy the diversions, challenges, and satisfactions that life has to offer.

"Waiting for that big city where the saints go marching in," suggests the hope for a positive afterlife once we leave this temporary mysterious place. To the extent that we can assume or believe that where we are going is positive or at least neutral, we calm the anxiety and fear built into our survival instinct.

"Life is like a mountain railway, with an engineer that's brave," suggests that courage is the desired attitude when dealing with challenges.

"If this is all there is to life, then I'll just keep on dancing," and "Rollin' with the flow" suggest a contented and graceful flow through the maze of life".

These sorts of positive attitudes and approaches to life and others like them can be found, explored, and cultivated both during psychedelic experience and during daily life.

A glimpse of the incredible magnificence and the miraculousness nature of creation in its wholeness that the high dose psychedelic experience can offer can also provide a greater peace of mind.

Seeing ourselves as very small parts of something of such grandeur can make our daily life difficulties seem much less significant.

Bringing new and useful concepts into our mental world can be as productive and satisfying as bringing new and useful objects into our material world.

Faith might be defined as believing something that has never been proved, but if it brings greater tranquility and peace of mind, it is certainly is not a sin.

Personal growth with or without the stimulation of psychedelic experience is a meaningful and satisfying lifestyle. It increases the quality of life.

In the long run, I think that psychedelics can help to move a person away from the mindset of a Scrooge McDuck frantically clawing at the world for nutrient to that of a Johnny Appleseed contentedly distributing positive time, energy, and resources to the world as he goes along.

An emotional feeling of an abundance of positive energy within oneself to be shared with the world through word and deed is certainly an improvement over a feeling of desperate sucking neediness to fill an inner void of insecurity. I believe that a chronic feeling of neediness is often due to an unnecessary excess of the hormones associated with the survival instinct and that they can be tamed through relaxation practice and meditation, psychedelic and otherwise. I believe also that there is a much more pleasant built-in inner attitude-emotion-concept that combines altruism, benevolence, compassion, charity, selflessness, and love and that it can be cultivated and expressed to the world; and that it can help to neutralize many personal mental and physical discomforts.

A flow of positive and constructive energy from the self to the outside world is a pleasure. It is good for mental health, it makes the world a better place, and it maximizes the likelihood of a return of positive circumstances. We tend to reap what we sow.

A mind at peace in a body trained to relax is a pleasure when times are good and a healthy, convenient, satisfying, and rational personal sanctuary when times are not so good.